STAYING FIT AFTER

40

(You're never too old to get fit and boost your health)

(2019)

By

Richard Robertson

You can also follow me here on Facebook

https://www.facebook.com/RichardRobertson40/

to stay updated with our latest news and new book releases

TABLE OF CONTENTS

INTRODUCTION

Quite often, people equate old age with frail body, deteriorating health and a general inability. An inability to be agile, to be fit and to pursue things that matters to a younger generation, sometimes, like staying healthy. Fortunately, the bulk of our beliefs as humans are wrong. Preserving your health is totally doable. While the body experiences shifts in metabolism as one ages, there are discernible ways to counter this dreadful aspect as the decades pass. In this book, we will explore common ways to remain fit as we approach midlife. Think deeply about your life. I'm sure you probably don't want to have an existential crisis right now, but really. If you're currently thirty-five, your life is probably heading in some direction, and it may not be a pretty one. I know people like to believe that age is just a number, but I'm here to break some unfortunate news to you. Your body will undergo some real changes, whether you want it to or not. The good news is you can develop a personal approach to these new changes and embrace them. You can absolutely ease the process by attaining healthy habits beforehand. It is never too late to change. Okay, so maybe you'll become slower, greyer, and weaker...but that can be delayed by several decades if you follow simple advice perfectly curated in this booklet. Can you imagine being forty, and being sharper, fitter, and healthier than you are now? I guarantee that you can achieve this.

You don't need to read this book from cover to cover. Instead use ***"Your Healthy Eating Check-ins"*** to assess your everyday food decisions and to find chapters and features that may relate to your own needs. Look for countless topics—in-depth features and brief snippets— that capture your interest: perhaps eating meatless meals sometimes or always; limiting food waste; exploring uncommon fruits, vegetables, and whole grains; shopping online or at a farmers' market; doing recipe makeovers; making simple shifts to healthier eating; helping a child grow or prepare food; eating for sports performance; taking supplements wisely; knowing more about pre- and probiotics; judging food experiences in child or adult day care; overcoming mindless eating; using today's mobile or digital health options; finding trustworthy eating advice; supporting healthy eating for others; and so much more, This comprehensive resource can help you take easy, practical, and flavourful steps toward your everyday healthy eating decisions and good health. From my table to yours, read, enjoy, be active, and eat healthy . . . for life!

CHAPTER 1

THE SCIENCE BEHIND AGING

Life happens too fast for too many people, leaving us little time to take care of ourselves while chasing the goodies of everyday living. A quick glance through the lives of an average forty-year old would most likely be a well-contrived chaos: you studied hard in college, and worked harder in your late twenties and early thirties. Got married, and tried every day for the next decade to juggle work, kids, spouse and paying debt together with having bits of fun and alone time. It's a crazy world. But that's all you've got. So by the time you're forty, you end up constantly worn-out, totally oblivious of the bad eating habits you've picked up over the years and the underlying health issues rising in the wake of your midlife. With so many illnesses, both treatable and untreatable. You do not have to exhaust yourself by searching for the fountain of Eden to achieve eternal youth. This book provides timeless, yet scientifically backed tips to staying young and healthy. One part is learning all the right foods to eat. You may have heard that the Mediterranean diet is the absolute best for anti-aging. We will explore what constitutes the Mediterranean diet, as well as what the average Japanese person eats throughout their life. We could learn a lot from the country which boasts the oldest average age for passing on. Then of course, there is exercise. Your body undergoes natural changes but with the right practice, these can be delayed. And finally, the psychological aspect of aging is immeasurable. You are above forty, you should own a jet and a billion dollar stashed away in your garage. Lies!

It's totally counter-intuitive but you need to stop spending so much money on anti-aging products. There's no secret miracle drug out there for you. Americans spend millions of dollars on these goose chases. Do you think you're less important, or a less valuable member of society by aging? No, you're not. Get your head out of the sand, and see the process of getting and remaining fit as a lifestyle choice. Enjoy the journey of it. You are what you think; you are what you eat; you are what you do.

All of this begs the question: What can you do? What will you do?

There is a saying that you cannot teach an old dog new tricks. Well, here's the good news: You're not a dog, and you're not old! You may not have the body of the top athletes in the world. Stop comparing yourself. Do you actually believe their lives are anything comparable to yours?

There are some terms we need to establish the definitions for before we proceed. You've probably heard the term thrown around a lot, from magic pills to supposed cancer-defying foods. Perhaps you're a little sceptical that it's even a real thing. Well, fortunately, it is a real thing, and yes it plays an extremely important role in maintaining health. Antioxidants do exist in the body and they're responsible for preventing a lot of harm. You might be surprised by the source of this harm - oxygen. Yeah, oxygen Oxidation of your cells is the primary source of aging. Certain foods contain antioxidants to offset the harm caused by oxidation. These foods will be explained later on.

Free radicals - what are they? Again, they probably sound a little conspiratorial and like some gimmick used to sell certain health supplements. Again, the term free radical is rooted in truth.

You may not remember how much energy you had during your twenties. That's okay. But know this, your hormones are responsible for the vast majority of this change, particularly for women. It's not all in your head, either. There's real science backing up why you feel so horribly. What are hormones, exactly? Well, they regulate a lot of aspects of the body, from hunger to libido to - you guessed it - metabolism. Which hormones exist in our bodies? It's different between men and women.

CHAPTER 2

EXERCISING IN OVER 40'S

Experts are of the opinion that, starting at the age of 40, we lose around 1% of our muscle strength each year, and by age 70, if unchecked, it may increase to 3 percent yearly. What this means is that by 80 years, we are so frail and without 60 percent of the strength we've garnered for a lifetime. Constantly losing muscle strength can affect your balance and increase your chances of falling. We all know that faking and losing balance can be quite fatal, resulting in hip fractures, and increasing the chance of early death. All of this can be drastically reduced, if we pay attention to the advice in this book. The simplest advice being: exercise daily. Suffice to say that your choice is obvious, when asked which to choose, exercising 30 minutes a day or gradually dying every hour of the day?

First Steps to Middle-Age Fitness

Starting a fitness routine can be overwhelming, especially if you've never done it before. But don't worry, as long as you start a work goal, and a commitment to stick with it, you are halfway there. You just have to keep reminding yourself that losing weight, getting stronger and improving your overall health is worth it. Next, check in with your doctor. Reason: the older you are, the greater your risk for medical conditions. Talk to your doctor about health conditions you have that may determine the best form of exercise for you. Have experts around to guide you, if you can, hire a personal trainer to help you achieve your goal and schedule your routine. People with trainers are far more likely to stick to their fitness routine.

Next, you need to build slowly. The goal is not to do a month's worth of exercise in a day. The key is gradual progression, and consistency. Note of advice, you're working out now, so your body is expected to react to the stress and pain. Don't be surprised then if you are sore, it's quite expected. Even as little work-out as a brisk work I'd expected to make you sore. But soreness to the point of not being able to move means you've overworked your body. Take it easy on yourself, after all, it's your first time. It is advisable to break your fitness routine to three segments of ten minutes apiece and interval to allow you rest at this To build overtime, you then gradually replace less rigorous physical activities like brisk walking with those that require more energy and rigour like jogging. You may find it useful to engage in interval training — intense spurs with regular intervals — which suggests that during brisk walk for instance, you speed for a while between street signs, then continue your normal pace for the next street sign. Repeating this process throughout your brisk walk will introduce a kind of regular strain and intensity to your exercise.

Your Guide to Good Health: Getting Specific

Cardiovascular exercises, strength training and flexibility training are three types of activities that must be featured in your fitness routine. While cardiovascular exercise focuses on your heart and lungs, strength training strengthens the muscles and ensures that muscle loss due to aging is at a minimal, and flexibility trailing helps preserve balance. For cardiovascular activities, basic exercises like biking, jogging, playing double tennis and brisk walking are effective for optimal results.

For strength training however, you need to work out once every two or three days, and never on consecutive days. Professional trainers are of the opinion that for these kinds of activities, it is the rest, and not the exercise itself, that matters. To get started, you begin with push-ups, squats, sit-ups and other whole body exercises. It will require you about three sets of ten repetitions to build your muscular strength and size in that part of your body, at least. More than free weights and weight machines, I suggest you use resistance bands because of their lower potential for injury.

How to Make Middle-Age Fitness Fun

More than anything, you should enjoy exercising. I know that's hardly your goal but it sure will help you maintain momentum and keep pushing. Having a workout buddy to exercise with is a good way to add fun to your work-out routine. Obviously, the person must be someone you're comfortable around, else, you end up not working out because you're avoiding the person. It is safe to make good friends, or partner your workout buddy. Your colleague at work is a no-no. Besides the people factor, you may want to engage in exercise that excites you. Some people like the idea of doing yoga while others like gardening. They both are effective work-out routines, the difference is your interest. Lastly, have a way to track your progress. Tracking your progress will give you a sense of accomplishment and make you enjoy exercising more.

CHAPTER 3

HOW TO WORK-OUT AS YOU AGE

Old age is never a fun thing, at least biologically. It limits the growth of muscle size and strength and exposes you to a lot of weaknesses, like having a lower recovery time. As if these were not enough, testosterone levels as well as bone quality decreases greatly as one ages, continually. And joint pains and aches become casual effects of bits of stressful endeavours. Changing your diet and engaging in some low impact sports and exercises are perfect solutions. As for exercise, it is recommended for all women between the ages of nineteen and sixty-four to receive a hundred and fifty minutes of moderate exercise each week in order to ward off diseases and increase body metabolism.

Cold scientific facts apart, at age forty, most of us would have been dealt a good blow by fate and lost more than once things we hold dear. With sense of loss comes frustration and other psychological problems. Imagine adding aging to all of the obvious loss accumulated over one's adult life, the pain would most likely be unbearable. Which is why you need to fight for those things you can still fight for, like your health. Instead of losing muscle size, with simple exercise and healthy routines, you can make gain over time.

You can reasonably gain a few pounds worth of muscle each month. It's better to start off the middle of your life with perhaps five, ten, possibly even fifteen more pounds worth of muscle than without it. Better yet, regular exercises will help you maintain that muscle for an extended period of time, too.

The workouts that I suggest are below with more following further down.

Overhead Press - Row aim for a low intensity, if the machine offers levels of resistance. Increase every two weeks by five percentages.

Bench Press - This might be a more advanced exercise but it is absolutely worth doing. Do four sets of three reps each.

Lunge - This might be a little more challenging, especially for those suffering from balance issues or knee problems.

Especially for those suffering from knee joint discomfort and pains, substitute this exercise for a leg press.

Back Extension - This is a great exercise to increase flexibility. It will also improve posture by strengthening your lower back muscles. However, do not arch your back so much that you become uncomfortable. It's otherwise an excellent exercise for toning your core as well as your back. You can customize these sample workouts but preferably with a qualified fitness trainer at your local gym. You can loosely follow the method of upping the strength by 5% every three weeks for increasing intensity. Your body will adapt and if you continue with the same workout it will be less effective. You want to aim for minimal breakdown of muscles but not too much that you become injured.

When exercising, avoid rapid movements. Do each exercise accurately, slowly, and under the auspices of a professional. You need a complete range of motions using a variety of muscles. Only doing push ups or sit ups will simply not be adequate. All workouts ought to be designed around using multiple joints and muscles as they mimic real life movements like climbing or walking on uneven and unsteady ground. If you do exercises intended to be done alone and to failure, you increase your risk for injury.

If you are interested in losing fat in a couple of weeks I'll introduce you to a perfect workout program just for that. As long as you are willing to do these workouts three or four times a week you're sure to lose fat. The following equipment is necessary to get you started: Barbell, Kettle Bell, DumbBells and anything that can help with cardio as well (treadmill, StairMaster or air dyne).

Loss of muscle, also known as muscle atrophy, is a major concern for people over the age of 40. Women in particular due to their physiological makeup have less bone density and muscle mass than men, and as such are more prone to muscle loss. However, baby boomers need to realize the importance of non-aerobic strength training for reducing muscle loss and preserving bones. For the first few weeks, do cardio for fifteen minutes only. Like one mile and a half. You'll burn approximately one hundred calories per mile. So, a hundred and fifty calories in fifteen minutes is actually pretty good. You can alternate between running and walking, too. This way you don't get overly exhausted right away. This workout is called HIIT. Actually, because you won't feel yourself being too tired, you'll probably be more inclined to stay on the treadmill a bit longer. You may initially only be able to run for no more than two minutes at 5 miles per hour. That's okay. Do this a couple of times, so long as the cardio in total for the first week reaches fifteen minutes.

For twenty minutes, engage in a couple of resistance training. Incline bench press is a great example, but be sure to have a spotter with you. Don't put on weight greater than forty pounds initially. Do three sets of ten reps each. Squats are highly recommended, provided you don't do them too rapidly. You'll work out your glutes, hamstrings, and core. Again, three sets of around eight to ten reps each is an excellent starting point. Start doing daily planks. Hold them in the beginning, in good form, for around a minute. Do three consecutive planks daily, and then increase by ten seconds every other week. The barbell row is an intense exercise, but be super careful about your form so you don't pull your back muscles.

The kettle bell looks simple, but don't be discouraged - it's actually one of the most intense workouts you can do. There are many ways to use it. I'll outline some of them here. For those who lack the means to invest in a monthly gym membership, the kettle bell is actually a great cardio and strength training workout combined. Moreover, the kettlebell still remains pretty under-rated, meaning that if your gym has any, they won't likely be monopolized by anyone.

The kettlebell swing is the standard exercise for all those who are first introduced to it. It is simple, as long as you use good form. To get started, stand with your feet at approximately the width of your shoulders. Bend over to pick up the kettle bell, but do not yank with your hands or else you will pull your back. When you lift it up ensure that you are using your whole body-weight to do so, and not just your arms. As you ascend, swing the kettlebell in front of you up to your neck while holding your arms straight with a slight bend at the elbow.

The kettlebell "goblet squats", while sounding like a scary Halloween move, is actually an excellent alternative to traditional squats. Start by holding the kettle bell to your chest.

The first position is in the squatting position. Then, ascend to full body length before squatting again. During this entire motion, you have the kettle bell held to your chest. Any squat move is amazing for fat burning potential. So, if every cardio machine happens to be occupied, this can be a quick substitute for it.

Dumbbells, on the other hand, are known for their versatility. They're an age old method for gaining muscle, specifically in your arms. Dumbbells are your best bet for inexpensive and mobile work-out equipment. Contrary to popular belief, even if you go light on the weight itself, (let's say you keep the weight around fifteen pounds only) you will still gain muscle. Choose a weight that sits between comfortable, but not excessively comfortable to carry. You do want to feel a little resistance. It's too heavy if you twist your back in order to be able to lift it.

There are lots of possible exercises to choose from. Choose one of these, I recommend you try them out first to determine which you find most comfortable:

Front Raise - This exercise is great for people without a lot of experience training. Stand upright with feet apart at the shoulders. With your arm extended, and legs apart, do a repetitive loft (weighing at least 10). Bring your arms from your thighs up to the height of your neck. To avoid muscle pull, don't yank the dumbbell. Instead, carefully work out your core little by little.

Overhead Press - Is another workout for the shoulders similar to the front raise. Here, however, you will keep your arms and the dumbbells parallel to your shoulders. Do not lock your elbows as this is dangerous and does not put stress on your muscles. Do it slowly, as you raise the dumb bells.

Barbells might be a little more advanced than your typical dumbbell or kettlebell arrangement. However, they're some of the most effective pieces of equipment at your gym for effective muscle gains. They're even considered to be better than dumbbells. By using the barbell, you are putting more strain on your muscles forcing them to tear and then rebuild.

The bench press is standard. It looks intimidating, and should be done next to a spotter. Especially at higher weights, don't do it alone! For this you need a bench. Lie down on your back with the barbell a few inches off your chest. Push above you without completely locking your elbow joints. Then, lower back down to a few inches off your chest again. Repeat this for about eight reps in three sets.

Do a variety of these workouts for each session, alternating between them to get a full body weekly workout. By keeping the weight a bit on the low side, but doing each movement more slowly, you will still maximize your gains compared to a normal speed with higher weights. While it sounds counter intuitive, you put more strain on your muscles as you hold them for longer. It isn't all about the weight. The goal is not to kill your muscles but to stimulate them. These workouts are going to be great to offset sarcopenia. **What exactly is that?**

Sarcopenia is the process of muscle loss as you age. As you lose muscle you will lose other functions slowly, as well. Such functions are balance, everyday motions of daily life (like picking up the morning newspaper or loading and unloading the dishwasher), and your manner of walking. It's a complex process that is mostly brought on by a sedentary lifestyle and poor nutrition. There is no medication approved for this condition, which means you need to adapt to a healthy lifestyle with plenty of exercise to stand a chance against it.

The Best Workout for People Over 40

DAYS	EXERCISE
Monday	Chest, Triceps
Tuesday	Rest
Wednesday	Back, Biceps
Thursday	Rest
Friday	Shoulder, Traps
Saturday	Rest
Sunday	Thigh, Calves, Abs

MONDAY

For days scheduled for chest/triceps workout, spend five minutes doing light cardio to get blood flowing through the body. Then your body will be ready for some 30 minute of moderate intensity cardio workouts. Stretch before and after workouts and make sure you have three minute rest periods between each set. Quantitatively do: ten slow Push Ups for warm-up. Three sets of Barbell Bench Press at 12, 12, 10 medium grip and two sets of Dumbbell Incline Bench Press at 12, 10. You can as well add two sets of Dumbbell Chest Flyes at 12, 8 be. Pretending to hug someone while exercising may help you get full range of motion.

Monday Safety tips:

Your elbows should be positioned away from your body. Make sure your hips are bent and your body is lowered till you feel a slight stretch at your heart. In order to stimulate your chest muscle you must push your body forward throughout the exercise. If you're doing barbell bench presses, you need to maximize chest stimulation by using a wide grip. Doing this will reduce your chances of injury while ensuring that momentum is on your side.

WEDNESDAY

On Wednesdays, make use of the middle back stretch technique. To do this, stand so your feet are shoulder width apart and your hands on your hips. Twist at your waist until you feel a stretch. Hold for 10-to-15 seconds, and then twist to the other side. You may as well add such exercises as standing torso reach and standing bicep stretch to make it more rigorous. Don't forget: rigorous is good. Quantitatively, on Wednesday you have to do ten assisted or free Pull Ups for warm-up, three sets of Lat Pull-Down at 12, 12, and two sets of Low Rows at 12, 8 keep the back as straight as possible. You may add two sets of High Rows at 12, 8 keep the back as straight as possible and three sets of Deadlifts at 12, 8 be sure to use excellent form.

Wednesday Safety Tips:

I will highlight the safety tips for using Alternating Dumbbell Curls and deadlift here. You only need these two for your

Wednesday exercise. For the former, keep your elbows as steady as possible. You may have to force the bicep to do most of the work of moving your weight. In order to maintain your proper form, don't swing your weight, instead lean back on a platform while lifting the dumbbells carefully. For the latter, try to keep your hips low, your shoulders should be high and arms straightened. Looking up at the ceiling may help you keep a proper form while you do this exercise.

FRIDAY

Shoulder/traps days involve side wrist pull, hands interlocked overhead and rear deltoid stretch. Side wrist pull for instance involves crossing your left arm over the midline of your body and holding the left wrist in your right hand down towards your hips. Feel free to stretch, bend and pull your shoulders while avoiding the temptation to switch sides.

Friday Safety Tips:

When doing this Side Dumbbell Lateral Raises, maintain elbows at an average of 20 degrees. Don't forget: shoulders are not raised by external rotation but by shoulder abduction.

Start off with the dumbbells to the side of the leg as opposed to in front of the leg, where momentum can be used. A mirror can come in handy when doing this to check it is lateral deltoids you are using and not anterior deltoids. For Dumbbell Rear Deltoid Raise, maintain your elbow still at 30 degrees or a minimum of 10 and ensure that your torso parallel to the floor. This will work the posterior deltoid instead of your lateral deltoid.

SUNDAY

On Sundays the focus is on thighs, calves and abs. Standing Quadriceps Stretch and Standing Hamstring Stretch are good examples of techniques that emphasize these thighs, abs and calves. Standing Quadriceps Stretch is simple. Handle one of your lower legs from behind. Force the lower leg toward your backside. Fix your hip by moving the knee in reverse. Hold the stretch and rehash with the other leg. For Standing Hamstring Stretch then again, you need to stand and twist around with the knees straight. Attempt to go after your toes or the floor. Your spine can either be kept straight or might be bowed.

Hold the stretch and rehash. Do fifteen free Squats for warm-up. Ensure you stretch your hamstrings to avoid damage.

Sunday Safety Tips:

When doing full hand weight squats, be certain that you keep your head forward, back straight and the two feet level on the floor. Ensure that the weight is similarly disseminated. While hunching down, ensure that the weight is circulated on your heels instead of your toes. Try not to bolt your knees after you complete every redundancy. For straight legged deadlift, start off with light loads to permit your body legitimate adjustment. Keep arms and knees straight all through this activity. Attempt to keep the free weight as near your body as could be allowed so you won't tilt over. In the event that you can't bring down the weight right to the floor, DON'T. Go until you feel a decent mellow stretch on your hamstrings before you go up. Full scope of movement may not be workable for a few.

Work-out Differences

As a forty-year old, your work-out plan should be somewhat different from that of a younger person, except if you're already an athlete and familiar with vigorous exercise routines. Your routine will be different because of health factors, motivation and other bodily limitations. Unlike younger people you'll meet at the gym, your muscle recovery wouldn't recover as quick as it used to and you are much increasingly more defenseless to damage over the long haul. Practically, when you hit the age of 40, your body begins deteriorating.

Not exclusively does your testosterone level abatements, your perseverance level and quality would be incredibly deteriorated. One of the most well-known issues among this age is osteoporosis. Osteoporosis is where the bone gets delicate because of the loss of bone thickness. When you arrive at a point where you are experiencing osteoporosis, it is difficult to turn around the procedure, subsequently the motivation behind why I can't stress enough about the significance of osteoporosis counteractive action.

Muscle decay would be another significant concern. Both of these procedures are unavoidable yet can be backed off with legitimate preparation. Once more, this is the place practicing takes care of later in your life. Indeed, having a decent body while you are youthful is a certain something, yet not experiencing back torments, muscle misfortune and having solid bones when you get more established would be another. Testosterone would need to be the most critical main factor between individuals beyond 40 years old, and the individuals younger than 40. As referenced previously, when you hit the age of 40, your body begins to neutralize you. As you get more established, your testosterone level begins to decay, and without testosterone, your body would not have the option to assemble more muscles. You are presently neutralizing a major detriment contrasted with the more youthful individuals. As the more youthful individuals work out, they have a high testosterone level which enables them to construct greater muscles at a quicker time frame. Individuals beyond 40 years old won't have this kind of advantage.

To wrap things up, injuries would undeniably be a boundary to many individuals more than 40. Older individuals are increasingly helpless to wounds because of the way that you just are not at your prime any longer. Your body can't persevere through all the extreme exercise that you were once ready to do.

Any sorts of strains, sprains and tissue harm towards the body will set aside a more extended time of effort to recuperate. Numerous individuals know about this reality and are not ready to go out on a limb. This should be a top need; in any case, it ought not get you far from revealing to yourself that you are never again fit to exercise.

Putting health factors aside, many people over 40 simply don't have enough time to work out. Because at this age, many people are now married and have to tend to their families and have workplace commitment.

Weakness could be a significant boundary averting individuals beyond 40 years old have a decent exercise. You will clearly be stressed out at work, and once you return home, it's a great opportunity to deal with the spouse and children. With all these, the urge to workout is minimal, if at all it exists. To correct this, you need to re-dedicate yourself to staying healthy.

Remind yourself why you're doing this in the first place: to stay healthy and make your older phase in life bearable. Thus, indicating the intrigue and responsibility will be the first and most significant advance you take to getting fruitful. If not, your body will continue deteriorating and more awful up to where it would be past the point of no return, in any event, when you show devotion.

CHAPTER 4

SUPPLEMENTS

You cannot work out a bad diet from your system. You'll need to refine your diet to include more whole foods and less processed crap, especially those marketed as healthy. I'd say eighty percent of all market foods are toxic trash that doesn't belong in anyone's kitchen. It might be unreasonable to expect you to read the fine details on every single product that you already have, but once you realize how companies sneak sugar into everything, the more fearful you will literally become when you go to the market. That is, unless you make the decision to cook your own foods using fresh, organic produce and makes protein the central focus of every meal.

Six packs are made in the kitchen, as the saying goes. You can do a zillion sit ups, crunches, whatever - but you will need to adjust your diet to have a low enough body fat percentage to show off those abs! Otherwise they're going to remain hidden from the entire world to see.

Contrary to popular belief, breakfast is not the most important meal of the day by any stretch of the imagination. We've all been told that growing up, but actually many people successfully skip breakfast and wait until lunch to start eating.

Intermittent fasting is highly recommended. What's that, you ask? Intermittent fasting is an age old technique used to cleanse the body and mind. Energy restriction - that is, keeping from consuming food between certain hours of the day - will restart your body and make you feel energized. The only catch is this: you cannot consume anything except for water and black coffee during the period of time established.

There are three popular kinds of intermittent fasting plans, a twelve-twelve orientation for eating. You eat during that half day window and then fast the other half. Others are eight-sixteen and twenty hours fasting! For the most committed among you, this will be fine. However don't start out with a twenty hour fast or you will go nuts.

There are other ways to accomplish intermittent fasting. For instance, you can do a 5:2 method - using this method, you eat normally for five days in the week but for two days you fast. You still eat, but only around five hundred to six hundred calories. If that's not OK with you, there's also the method called Eat-Stop-Eat. With this method, you eat normally all week, but for one day you stop eating for a twenty four period of time. This is not a beginner's fast!

OMAD - One Meal a Day - as suggested, eat once per day. Be careful, though. This does not work for everyone. Don't just load up on beer and burgers and call it a meal. You need to ensure that your one meal takes care of all your nutrient needs.

Your body and brain will benefit a lot from fasting. When you consider the fact that during the first millennia of human history, people didn't have fast food joints or supermarkets readily available to them, so they had to fast. Our bodies are still built to roam the Savannah. We hunted in tribes, finding food and feasting, then going another few days with no food until the next kill. Our bodies learned to thrive under these dire conditions. However our lives are nothing like that anymore -

we mostly lead sedentary lives in which we expect food to be put in front of us three times a day.

How to start an intermittent fasting diet? It sounds a lot easier than it actually is. Just stop eating, right? Well, no. You still need to ensure that you're getting all the nutrients you need. If you elect to a diet in which you have a six hour or eight hour window to eat, eat normally but only during that single timeframe for eating. The logic goes that you'll be naturally eating less, as long as you don't compensate by shovelling food down your throat.

A basic framework for good nutrition is as follows:

- ☐ Try to aim for full fat yogurt and other dairy products. This might seem counter intuitive, however lower fat or fat free yogurts have a tendency to include more sugar to make up for less fat, which offers flavour. More unfortunately is the common tendency for companies to market products as fat free only to add starch or other thickeners to improve consistency. This obviously has excessive carbs that are not healthy!

- ☐ Go green! Get big leafy greens for vegetables as they contain a lot of iron and other necessary nutrients.

- ☐ Protein is your friend! You need to make protein account for the larger chunk of your meal. Eggs or sausage for breakfast, chicken or turkey for lunch, and then more chicken or another kind of meat or fish for dinner. If you're not a big fan of meat, that's understandable. You can substitute beans to a certain extent. Also, lentils are an excellent source of protein as well.

- ☐ There are healthy oils. Olive oil is an excellent choice. A close second would be coconut oil.

On a final note, besides a healthy meal, the only thing worth talking about is supplement. While they are not a substitute for a healthy meal, they however are very useful for people over forty who are interested in leading a healthy life. Vitamin D3 for instance is important for deficiency in Vitamin D, since many people over the age of forty are most likely receiving very little exposure to sun due to work. Women over forty especially need to be careful that they are receiving enough

Vitamin D because the lack of it causes, among other things, hair loss, fatigue and frequent bouts of depression.

Omega 3 is another good supplement. Usually derived from fish oils, it supplements the lack of fat in one's body. While fat carries a negative reputation, in pop culture, some fat is critical for literal brain function. Enough Omega 3s can reduce your risk for various diseases, especially those pertaining to memory and weight loss. Omegas 3 are shown to also reduce the risk for high cholesterol, certain kinds of cancer, macular degeneration, and arthritis. It is not recommended to have a diet completely free from all animal products if you cannot reasonably consume enough plant sources of Omega 3s, since fish is the absolute best natural food for it.

Magnesium is another worrisome issue for those past the age of forty. Magnesium levels must be adequate, this is because over three hundred of our body functions rely on appropriate amounts of Magnesium. Magnesium deficiency is a common problem for people with unhealthy diets. There are many lesser known reasons for deficiency - for instance, frequent consumption of coffee may inhibit magnesium absorption. If you are on heart medicine or a diuretic (which is a medicine that encourages more frequent urination) then magnesium deficiency is a very common side effect. It is recommended to take a combination supplement of calcium and magnesium to encourage more absorption of both. Magnesium deficiency is dangerous. While some symptoms are more annoying than anything, such as frequent migraines, impotence, and insomnia, others pose a more dangerous health risk. Osteoporosis, bacterial infections, kidney or liver damage, incapacitating PMS symptoms, and tooth cavities all become more common problems among people lacking enough Magnesium. Magnesium Citrate is the easiest to absorb of all Magnesium supplements while other dietary supplements like HMB (Beta-hydroxy-beta-methyl butyrate) have shown the potential to assist in building muscle, particularly for lean individuals who are just beginning a regime.

Multi Vitamins: Perhaps the most important supplement. Multivitamin should be taken by everybody, but especially those people who work out often like us. The reason is that our body is constantly expending energy and thus we lose lots of vitamins and minerals.

For those over 40, I recommend taking multivitamins. High dosages of vitamins are not necessary. A simple multivitamin should do.

Protein Powder: Muscle heads commonly expend 1.5-2 grams of protein for each bodyweight. It is essential to expend in any event one gram of protein for each body weight to manufacture and fortify muscles. Genuine nourishment high in protein should start things out. Nourishments like steak, chicken, fish and fish are high in protein. Notwithstanding, it's not possible for anyone to expend that much protein as far as unadulterated nourishment. That is the place where protein powder becomes an integral factor. Proteins are the fundamental structure squares required to fabricate muscles. There are two sorts of protein, the first being whey protein (quick acting proteins that experience your whole body in an hour or less. They are normally taken when exercises to construct and fix muscles) and casein protein (slow-processing sort of protein. They can take as long as 5 hours to experience the whole human body. They are regularly taken before bed to keep the body from heading off to a catabolic state).

Milk: Milk is very good for your body. Not only does it contain 35 percent calcium, it also contains 25 percent Vitamin D. Which means it helps in both mental health and bodily strength as well. I encourage you to mix your protein shake with milk, that way, you have 3 to 4 glasses of milk per day and a higher concentration of protein in your system. Remember, the road to a healthy diet is paved with protein.

Glucosamine: By now, you already know and have made your peace with the fact that older people are more prone to health problems. Basic joint pain can greatly disturb you from working out. It is this incessant joint pain that glucosamine eradicates.

Natural Testosterone Boosters:

Remember that we talked about testosterone earlier and how it affects your work-out results as you grow older. Without testosterone, your body cannot build muscles. Notwithstanding how hard you are working out. Indeed, there's a route around that. Everybody, who turns out necessities is a mind boggling source of multivitamins. What's more, I would state that over 40 Vitamin A, Vitamin

C, Vitamin D and extra calcium are the most common enhancements to upgrade vitality. For your post exercise dinner includes around 1 tablespoon of glutamine and creatine since it expands the hydration condition of the muscle cells.

CHAPTER 5

MENTALITY

Let's get one thing straight: Forty isn't old, and if you're thinking that way, you're already way behind. You shouldn't compare yourself with your all-time best. Instead, compare yourself with the average guy at your age. You have to set a higher standard than the norm, trust me, being normal sucks.

Step 1 – Mentally Prepare Yourself For Success.

You have to believe you're going to succeed in your goal of getting in shape at 40. Without this drive you will still struggle to develop healthy habits and lifestyle changes that are essential to finding the new you. You can only achieve what you have imagined.

Step 2 – Give Yourself A Bedtime.

You may have thought that you no longer need a bedtime; this is something that you do for children to ensure they get enough sleep, (or to make sure you have an evening). However, you need to get at least 6 or 7 hours of sleep a night. The best way to achieve this is to fix your sleep schedule and set yourself a bedtime. Instead of focusing on the next film, regardless of what time it ends, know that you need to go to bed. Of course, you should ask why getting to bed on time matters for getting into shape. Other than possibly giving you an energy boost it may not feel that important. But it is! When you sleep, your body balances your hormone levels. Ghrelin levels decrease when you sleep. As this is the hormone that tells your body when you are hungry, lower levels are good! At the same time sleeping increases your levels of leptin, which is the hormone that tells your body you have had enough to eat. In this case, higher levels are what you need.

Step 3 – **Plan, Prepare and Pack Your Meals.**

The Fit Father Project has planned a scope of supper plans for you to test. It will outline the sorts of nourishment you ought to eat and that it is so natural to alter your dietary patterns.

The initial step, which you can take at the present time, is to stop eating handled nourishment. Try not to endeavor to do this only for you; think about your family also. Like I said before, the enormous lump of nourishment Americans eat dangerous garbage! Once more, quit eating prepared nourishment. Search for savvy approaches to checkmate your utilization of these nourishment and void your cooler of them.

Step 4 – Start Walking.

Albeit good dieting will have the greatest impact on getting fit as a fiddle at 40, you do in any case need to work out, or if nothing else perform physical activity each day. Strolling for thirty minutes every day can have a significant effect in the blink of an eye. Working is the incredible decision for you, if like you're in every case too occupied to even consider working out. You can decide to drive by walking rather than the vehicle, stroll at mid-day break or even before anything else. The significant thing is to manufacture a propensity for this basic movement. It is the foundation of having sufficient opportunity to present progressively serious and profitable exercise. There is a basic explanation behind this: activity expands the degree of fit muscle in your body. Muscle consumes a bigger number of calories than fat. Along these lines, the higher your muscle (and lower your fat), the more calories you can expend without putting on weight. This does not mean that on the off chance that you practice you can eat what you like!

Step 5 – Build A More Intense Workout.

In your journey to being more healthy, many websites, apps and friends will hate you unsolicited advice regarding the best workout you should do. While some of them may be good for you, not all will be.

Luckily, by following these rules, you will. Just supplant your ongoing stroll with the Fit Father 24-min fat consuming exercise. This exercise, alongside the numerous others that you can access through the Fit Father Project, can be accomplished in under thirty minutes! It is around high-force practices that produce the greatest outcomes in the negligible conceivable time; enabling you to open it effectively into your bustling timetable and join the a large number of other men more than

40 who have added getting fit as a fiddle to their accomplishments; even past 40 or 60!

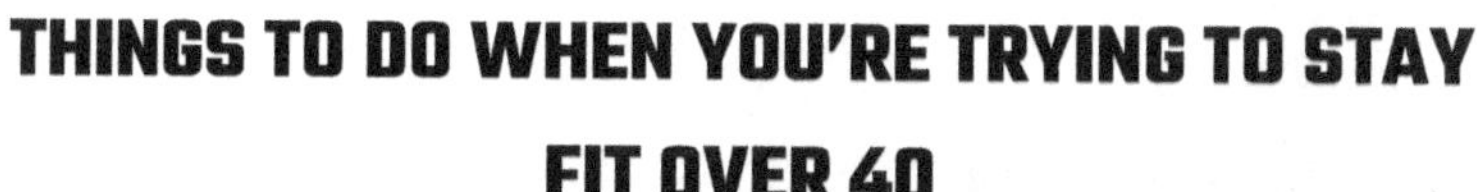

CHAPTER 6

THINGS TO DO WHEN YOU'RE TRYING TO STAY FIT OVER 40

1. Try not to let your digestion moderate down — Do BURPEES.

High-force cardio invigorates our metabolism, which is more than would normally be appropriate to motivate after a certain age. To prevent digestion deceleration, we should do this practice once or twice every week. Start with one set of 3 reps and include another reiteration each time. Try not to push yourself to an extreme.

2. Keep it firm —Do SQUATS.

Each lady needs to have a round rear yet even the most fortunate ones who had it naturally with no preparation will begin to lose it after the age of 40 thanks to the decline of muscle mass. Properly done squats (with a straight back and knees directly over the feet) can condition your entire body and forestall damage by improving your adaptability.

3. To fight and avoid back pain —Do a PLANK.

Doing this activity for 90 seconds 3 times a week is a great way to tone all the muscles of our bodies. It strengthens our abs, the muscles of the chest, and the ones encompassing the spine, our whole midriff fixes and supports our lower back.

4. Shield yourself from arthritis —Push DUMBBELLS.

Constant joint pain is a typical sickness among grown-ups, so it's never too early to start anticipating it and one of the most ideal ways to do it is strength preparation. You don't have to spend hours lifting huge loads. Doing deadlifts or overhead presses with 1-3 kg in each hand 2-3 times a week can do miracles for your body. By following the format given in this book, you can incredibly decrease your odds of getting this interminable disease.

5. Let your glutes rest —Do a GLUTE BRIDGE.

Sitting throughout the day in an office can deactivate our glutes which hinders the rate at which our body consumes calories —the digestion. The hip expansion in the glute bridge exercise makes the butt work and it can likewise open up any snugness from long days of sitting. Leave your arms along your sides, press your butt muscles to lift your hips up, and crush them again at the top, and afterward gradually let your hips down.

6. Try not to let sarcopenia take your muscles away — Do Y-TO-T RAISES.

Sarcopenia is a degenerative misfortune of skeletal muscle related to maturing. If you'd like to prevent awful stances and back and shoulder throbs, it is very significant to strengthen the muscles of your back and shoulders.

7. Secure your heart —Train on an ELLIPTICAL MACHINE.

Low-sway cardio is a great path for ladies over 40 to maintain a healthy heart. In any case, if you truly need your heart wellbeing to benefit, you need to exercise at 80% of your most extreme pulse for at least 30 minutes, 3 to 4 times a week. If 10 is as hard as you can do on a scale of one to 10, at that point you should work at the level of 8.

8. Live actively —WALK.

Strolling is the easiest and the best exercise that anybody can do. While it burns calories, conditions our body, and improves our state of mind, it also doesn't wear out our delicate joints, which is very significant after a certain age.

9. Relax —Do YOGA.

Moderately aged ladies are increasingly inclined to becoming discouraged, concurring to John Hopkins Medicine, one of the driving human services frameworks in the United States. Yoga increases a mood-managing synapse, which is necessary to fight melancholy. It also diminishes pressure and uneasiness levels.

CONCLUSION

This book has condensed information about the science of one's body, appropriate workouts, diet, and nutrition. The aim was to provide a concise overview as to inspire readers such as you to go and pursue it further. Take the information, keep it in the back of your mind, and build on it. Older men and women can still build muscle. The biggest takeaway you should have from reading this is that with age you do not have to compromise on health. I'd say that approaching health while aging requires extra care and understanding, since two things are happening - the physical loss of the body, and the mental realization that you, at some point, may not be able to accomplish the things you want to accomplish anymore. But, by following this advice, you can approach the age and endure it with a healthier outlook. One last thing that I will mention is how this will affect your mood. It's proven that a healthier diet entails a healthier attitude, and therefore a healthier philosophy toward life. You'll benefit from this enormously. As you can imagine, approaching the inevitable latter decades of one's life takes serious guts. It's going to be a journey, and it best is one with the healthiest body, mind, and spirit possible. Excessive added sugar is known to make one feel sluggish, so why do the counterproductive thing by downing milkshake after milkshake? Quit the nihilistic attitude and start taking care of yourself. You deserve to live out the remainder of your life with as much dignity as possible. As should be obvious, individuals beyond 40 years old make some harder memories having powerful exercises, yet it is not even close to outlandish. It merits the little extra difficult work, since it will pay off as you get more established. There are numerous kinds of issues as you get more seasoned, and a portion of the more typical ones would incorporate the loss of muscle size, also called muscle decay, just as the misfortune in bone thickness, also called osteoporosis. Presently except if individuals wouldn't fret having delicate bones and no quality as they get more established, everybody, particularly individuals beyond 40 years old should investigate having to some degree a powerful exercise. On the off chance that you can pursue the exercise schedule, have appropriate sustenance, and take a couple of enhancements to help support your exhibition, at that point you are headed toward a sound and cheerful life. Presently, obviously, as you get more established, you can't stop the procedure of muscle decay and osteoporosis, yet you can even now defer it. That ought to be an adequate impetus for everybody beyond 40 years old to begin turning out once more. At long last, it's so critical to make a mind-blowing most and feel great in the body you've been given and the most ideal approach to appreciate a long life is to eat well and exercise normally.

The End

Thanks for taking the time to read my book. I hope it helped you out in some type of way. If you are not already please go now and follow me here on fb at

https://www.facebook.com/RichardRobertson40/ .

By following me you will receive updates on all of my upcoming books, giveaways, also you will be the first to get free copies of all of my books.

Never miss another update

You can also follow me here on my Author's Page on Amazon.

Just Because

Just because you took the time to read my book here are two of my Keto Diet Books **FREE**. Sign up and get your books.

The guide to staying healthy after 40 for women...The Keto way

The guide to staying healthy after 40 for men...The Keto way